SCIENCE
OF
VITAMIN A

EVERYTHING YOU NEED TO KNOW ABOUT VITAMIN A

LA FONCEUR

Eb
emerald books

Eb

emerald books

Copyright © 2024 La Fonceur

All rights reserved.

No part of this publication may be reproduced, stored in a retrieval system or transmitted in any form or by any means, electronic, mechanical, photocopying, recording or otherwise, without prior permission of author.

Cover illustration by Famenxt

This book has been published with all efforts taken to make the material error-free. The information on this book is not intended or implied to be a substitute for diagnosis, prognosis, treatment, prescription, and/or dietary advice from a licensed health professional. Author and publisher don't assume and hereby disclaim any liability to any party for any loss, damage, or disruption caused by errors or omissions, whether such errors or omissions result from negligence, accident, or any other cause.

While every effort has been made to avoid any mistake or omission, this publication is being sold on the condition and understanding that neither the author nor the publishers or printers would be liable in any manner to any person by reason of any mistake or omission in this publication or for any action taken or omitted to be taken or advice rendered or accepted on the basis of this work. Some contents that are available in electronic books may not be available in print, or vice versa.

CONTENTS

Introduction   5

Chapter 1: Everything You Need to Know About
Vitamin A   7

Chapter 2: Importance of Vitamin A   21

Chapter 3: 10 Best Foods Rich in Vitamin A   38

Chapter 4: Potentially Dangerous Vitamin A
Combinations You Should Avoid   47

Chapter 5: Vitamin A Combinations for Synergistic
Health Benefits   50

Chapter 6: Diet Plan   54

Chapter 7: Recipes   56

    Pan Fried Cheesy Mushrooms   *57*

    Stuffed Bell Pepper   *59*

    Sarso Ka Saag   *62*

Read the Eat So What! Series   65

References   66

Contents

About the Author   **77**

Read More from La Fonceur   **78**

Connect with La Fonceur   **78**

Color Your Vitamin A   **78**

INTRODUCTION

The term "vitamin" is often thrown around. While we may have some knowledge regarding vitamins, do we really know all about vitamins? While we may have some vitamin knowledge, our awareness is often limited to what we hear from health advocates or simply dietary supplement manufacturing companies. You may come across countless articles promoting the benefits of vitamins, and they often conclude with recommendations for specific supplements.

Supplements have become easily accessible and convenient, saving time and effort. Many rely on supplements due to a busy lifestyle and limited knowledge about what their body needs for optimal health. This dependence may stem from fear or a reluctance to put in the effort to obtain necessary nutrients.

There are many misleading approaches available in the market. It is important to have accurate information because half-baked knowledge can be more harmful than no knowledge at all. Vitamin supplements may be beneficial, they are not regulated by the FDA, and overdose is common and dangerous. Unless your doctor has prescribed a supplement for a medical condition or deficiency, it is best to rely on whole foods to meet your nutrient needs.

Vitamins have been known to affect your health in numerous ways, some of which are yet to be fully discovered. This is why relying on vitamin supplements may not provide the same results that can be effortlessly obtained through natural sources. If you're not focusing on getting your necessary vitamins from food, you're missing out on a lot of potential health benefits.

You will get all the answers about fat-soluble Vitamin A in the ***The Science of Vitamin A*** book. Learn about vitamin A crucial role in maintaining good health and the latest scientific findings and how these can affect your vitamin decisions. Clear up common vitamin A related dilemmas, such as how to tell if you're deficient in vitamin A and when to get tested.

Learn about the advantages of combining vitamin A with other vitamins and foods for optimal health benefits, as well as the potential consequences of taking certain vitamin A with particular foods or medications. This guide covers both beneficial and harmful combinations of vitamin A, as well as the advantages and drawbacks of vitamin A supplement.

Furthermore, learn about nutrient-rich vegetarian options that are high in vitamin A. By consuming these foods, you can avoid vitamin A deficiencies and maintain good overall health, reducing the likelihood of infections and chronic illnesses such as cancer, diabetes, high blood pressure, and cognitive decline. Plus, explore some nutritious and easy-to-cook vegetarian recipes that can be included in your diet to maximize the health benefits of vitamin A.

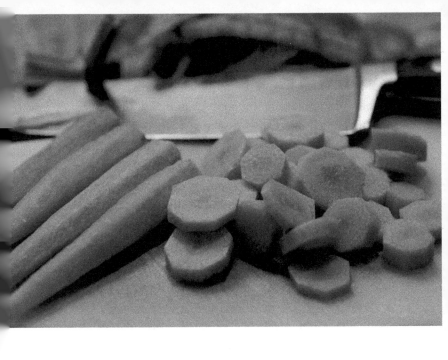

CHAPTER 1

EVERYTHING YOU NEED TO KNOW ABOUT VITAMIN A

Vitamin A, also known as retinol, is an essential fat-soluble vitamin found in both plant-based foods and animal-sourced products. It plays a vital function in growth and development, reproduction, immune function, and eye health. Vitamin A plays a vital role in the growth and differentiation of cells, contributing significantly to the proper development and maintenance of vital organs like the heart, eyes, lungs, and other organs.

What are carotenoids?

Fruits and vegetables get their bright yellow, orange, and red colors from pigments called carotenoids. Some examples of produce containing carotenoids include mangoes, papayas, bell peppers, carrots, and tomatoes. The most common types of carotenoids are beta-carotene, alpha-carotene, beta-cryptoxanthin, lutein, lycopene, and zeaxanthin.

How are carotenoids related to Vitamin A?

Your body has the ability to convert certain carotenoids into Vitamin A. Some examples of these carotenes include beta-carotene, alpha-carotene, and beta-cryptoxanthin.

Types of Vitamin A

Preformed Vitamin A (Animal-based Vitamin A)

As the name suggests, this type of Vitamin A is already made and found in animal products. Preformed Vitamin A (retinol and retinyl esters) is found in dairy products, fortified foods, and vitamin supplements (as retinyl palmitate or retinyl acetate).

Provitamin A Carotenoids (Plant-based Vitamin A)

Provitamin A carotenoids or precursors to Vitamin A are naturally present in fruits and vegetables. Your body converts Provitamin A carotenoids into Vitamin A in your intestine. Beta-carotene is the most common Provitamin A carotenoid present in foods and vitamin supplements.

Non-Provitamin A Carotenoids: Other carotenoids present in food, such as lycopene, lutein, and zeaxanthin, are non-Provitamin A carotenoids and are not converted to Vitamin A in the body but have other vital functions in the body.

How much Vitamin A do I need in a day?

The amount of Vitamin A in food is measured in micrograms (μg) of retinol activity equivalents (RAE). To fulfill the Vitamin A needs of healthy people, the recommended daily intake is:

Age	RDAs for Vitamin A (mcg RAE)	
	Male	Female
0 to 12 months*	400 mcg RAE	400 mcg RAE
1–8 years	300 mcg RAE	300 mcg RAE
9–13 years	600 mcg RAE	600 mcg RAE
14–50+ years	900 mcg RAE	700 mcg RAE

*Adequate Intake (AI)

Adequate intake is the level considered to ensure nutritional adequacy when there is insufficient evidence to develop Recommended Dietary Allowances.

1 mcg RAE is = 1 mcg retinol = 12 mcg dietary beta-carotene = 24 mcg dietary alpha-carotene or beta-cryptoxanthin.

Vitamin A doesn't need to be consumed daily. Your body stores extra Vitamin A for future use, meaning if you consume 2-3 mangoes a day, your body will convert beta carotene into Vitamin A and use up the daily required amount while storing the rest for later. Vitamin A is stored in your liver in the form of retinyl esters, like retinyl palmitate. Preformed Vitamin A, or retinyl ester, is converted into retinol after absorption in the lumen, and Provitamin A carotenoids are converted to retinol after absorption. In your body, retinol is oxidized into retinal and retinoic acid, the two main active metabolites of Vitamin A.

Is Provitamin A better than Preformed Vitamin A?

Preformed Vitamin A is better absorbed by the body than beta-carotene but is toxic at high levels. This is more common with preformed Vitamin A supplements and requires monitoring of intake levels. Another drawback is that too much preformed Vitamin A can interfere with the beneficial actions of vitamin D. Also, high levels of it may increase the risk of bone loss, hip fractures, or certain birth defects.

On the other hand, there is no such problem with beta-carotene. Your body can make as much Vitamin A as it needs from beta-carotene, and consuming high levels of beta-carotene is not toxic, so there is no need to monitor intake levels. Although consuming excessive amounts of beta-carotene can cause the skin to turn yellow-orange, this condition is harmless and goes away when you consume less of it. Additionally, beta-carotene acts as an antioxidant and has various positive effects on overall health. Beta carotene may offer you protection against various chronic diseases. Therefore, it is more beneficial to take Vitamin A in the form of beta-carotene.

But too much of anything is not good for health, so consume beta carotene in moderation and get it through food, not dietary supplements. Avoid higher-dose beta-carotene supplements as they may do more harm than good. People with hypothyroidism cannot convert beta-carotene into Vitamin A effectively, and this can be a problem. Studies have also shown that people who smoke or are exposed to asbestos and take beta-carotene supplements of high-dose may have a higher risk of lung cancer and death. So, keep in mind moderation is the key to health.

Does cooking affect the amount of Vitamin A in food?

The body can absorb preformed Vitamin A better than beta carotene. Preformed Vitamin A in the form of retinol can get absorbed about 75% to 100% in the body, and approximately 10% to 30% of beta-carotene from foods are absorbed in the body, but beta-carotene has other important function, such as killing the free radicals in the body. So, despite a low absorption rate, keeping your diet full of beta carotene can have various yet to be discovered health benefits. One way to increase the absorption of beta-carotene from foods is to cook them. Cooking helps release more beta-carotene from food, but it is most effective when you are roasting or baking the food. Boiling for long or stir-frying may result in a 10-15% loss of beta carotene. So, make sure not to boil the food for long or in lots of water to prevent the leaching of beta-carotene in water.

Another way to increase beta-carotene absorption in your body is to cook beta-carotene foods in oil or eat them with other healthy fats, as Vitamin A is a fat-soluble vitamin, and it needs the presence of fat in the body to get properly absorbed.

Is it dangerous to be low in Vitamin A?

Vitamin A is an essential vitamin that your body needs to function properly, and you must get it from food. If you are low in Vitamin A, it can affect many organs, such as the eyes, skin, heart, and reproductive organs. It also affects the defense system of your body against illness. Long-term Vitamin A deficiency can even lead to blindness.

What can happen if I have a Vitamin A deficiency?

Vitamin A deficiency or hypovitaminosis A can be the cause of several disorders. If you are deficient in Vitamin A, you are predisposed to the following conditions:

Eye Problems: Your eyes depend on vitamin A for many vital functions. Vitamin A deficiency can affect overall eye health. The early sign of vitamin A deficiency is difficulty seeing in low light, also known as night blindness. If this deficiency persists over a long period, a person may develop xerophthalmia, a condition where the cells in the cornea change, causing corneal ulcers, lesions, and eventually blindness.

Prone to Infections: Vitamin A is an essential vitamin for your immune system. It helps enhance immune function and plays a crucial role in the development of the immune system and immune responses. Vitamin A regulates the differentiation of immune cells that are necessary for immune tolerance throughout adult life. If you lack Vitamin A, it can impair the function of neutrophils, macrophages, natural killer cells, and T-cell mediated antibody responses, leading to decreased protective mechanisms. Additionally, a deficiency in Vitamin A can reduce mucus production, which increases the risk of invasive pathogens. Vitamin A has therapeutic effects on various infectious digestive diseases, particularly in children, such as diarrhea and hand, foot, and mouth disease.

Infertility: Sufficient intake of Vitamin A is vital for reproduction in both men and women, as well as for several processes during the development of the fetus. Insufficient Vitamin A intake can make it more challenging to get pregnant and result in infertility.

Retard Growth in Children: Vitamin A is essential for growth and development. For children, adequate Vitamin A status is more critical. Vitamin A deficiency contributes to retarded growth in children with persistent diarrhea.

Skin Problems: Vitamin A is essential for reducing inflammation and maintaining healthy skin. If your body lacks Vitamin A, you may be more prone to experiencing skin issues such as eczema and acne. Additionally, a deficiency in Vitamin A can result in hyperkeratosis, a skin condition where the outer layer of your skin, composed of keratin, becomes thicker than normal.

Respiratory Diseases: Not getting enough Vitamin A can increase your risk of chronic respiratory diseases like chronic obstructive pulmonary disease, pulmonary fibrosis, emphysema, and lung cancer. It can also make you more vulnerable to asthma due to higher susceptibility to oxidative stress. In young children under five years old, low Vitamin A levels are strongly linked to respiratory diseases. Babies and toddlers who lack Vitamin A are at a higher risk of severe respiratory infections like pneumonia, childhood asthma, and measles.

Thyroid Dysfunction: Severe Vitamin A deficiency is associated with a higher risk of goiter and high concentrations of circulating thyroid stimulating hormone (TSH) and thyroid hormones. Vitamin A deficiency interferes with the pituitary thyroid axis. Lack of enough Vitamin A in the body can lead to increased production and secretion of thyroid-stimulating hormone (TSH) by the pituitary gland. It also increases the size of the thyroid gland and reduces iodine uptake by the thyroid gland. Iodine deficiency often co-exists with Vitamin A deficiency. Concurrent iodine deficiency and Vitamin A deficiency produce more severe primary hypothyroidism than iodine deficiency alone.

Anemia: Anemia is a global health issue that can be caused by various factors, including a lack of Vitamin A. Vitamin A helps the body use iron more effectively. It also influences the growth and development of red blood cells and supports iron absorption by forming a complex with nonheme iron. Insufficient Vitamin A intake can lead to abnormal red blood cell shapes, causing microcytic or hypochromic anemia. This type of anemia is characterized by smaller than usual red blood cells (microcytic) with reduced red color (hypochromic) and increased iron storage in the liver. Vitamin A deficiency also reduces the transportation of iron in the body. Treating this type of anemia with iron supplements is ineffective, so Vitamin A supplements are necessary.

Also read: 10 Power Foods to Prevent Anemia in the Book Eat So What! The Power of Vegetarianism.

Weaker Bones: Vitamin A deficiency increases the risk of fractures. Adequate Vitamin A intake (900 mcg for men and 700 mcg for women) is essential for building strong and healthy bones. Vitamin A influences both osteoblasts (bone-building cells) and osteoclasts (bone-breaking down cells). Provitamin A (beta-carotene and beta-cryptoxanthin) protects bones. However, high Vitamin A levels, especially in conjunction with vitamin D deficiency, have been associated with decreased bone density and increased fractures.

What are the causes of Vitamin A deficiency?

There can be various factors that can cause Vitamin A deficiency. The most common reason is due to poor diet, but other factors like disease conditions can also lead to Vitamin A deficiency. Let's see the reasons one by one:

Poor Diet: A diet that lacks Vitamin A-rich foods or inadequate intake of Vitamin A required for physiological needs can cause Vitamin A deficiency in the body.

Fat Malabsorption: Fat malabsorption is a disorder in which your body is unable to absorb fat from your diet. This disorder can be caused by disruptions in your digestion process, including bacterial infection, inadequate digestive enzymes, or faster bowel movements than normal. As Vitamin A is a fat-soluble vitamin, fat malabsorption can affect the absorption of

Vitamin A in your body, which can result in Vitamin A deficiency despite consuming a diet rich in Vitamin A.

Certain Disease Conditions: Certain disease conditions, such as impaired pancreatic or biliary secretion, as well as inflammatory bowel diseases like celiac disease and Crohn's disease, can also cause fat malabsorption and hinder Vitamin A absorption in the body, leading to a deficiency of this important nutrient.

Zinc Deficiency: Zinc is crucial for transporting vitamin A in the body. If your diet lacks zinc, it won't impact the absorption or transportation of Vitamin A to the liver. However, it will restrict your body's ability to transfer Vitamin A from the liver to the body tissues. This may result in Vitamin A deficiency.

Iron Deficiency: Iron deficiency can cause Vitamin A to accumulate in the liver, resulting in reduced plasma retinol concentrations. This can negatively affect the mobilization of Vitamin A from the liver and ultimately decrease plasma retinol concentration, depriving you of the health benefits of Vitamin A.

How do I know if I am deficient in Vitamin A?

The symptoms of Vitamin A deficiency are as follows:

Night Blindness: One of the early indicators of vitamin A deficiency is night blindness, which is when you experience difficulty seeing in low-light conditions but have normal vision in well-lit areas.

Hazy Vision: Another symptom is hazy vision, which is caused by the buildup of keratin in the eyes, known as Bitot's spots. This occurs due to a lack of Vitamin A in the body.

Skin Diseases: If you're experiencing skin problems, you may want to consider whether you're getting enough Vitamin A in your diet. Vitamin A is essential for repairing skin cells. When your body doesn't have enough of this Vitamin, your skin can become dry, scaly, and inflamed, leading to conditions like eczema and acne.

Respiratory Infections: Vitamin A is important for a healthy immune system, and a deficiency in this Vitamin can make you more susceptible to respiratory infections in your chest and throat.

Infertility: Maintaining adequate levels of Vitamin A is crucial for the proper functioning of both male and female reproductive systems. A deficiency in vitamin A can lead to difficulties in conceiving and infertility.

Delayed Growth: Insufficient intake of Vitamin A can result in slow growth or delayed bone growth, leading to stunted growth in children.

Poor Wound Healing: Vitamin A plays a vital role in enhancing the production of collagen type I and fibronectin, which can increase the rate of wound closure and restore the skin structure. If you have low levels of Vitamin A, wounds may not heal properly after injury or surgery.

What should I do if I have Vitamin A deficiency symptoms?

You should consult your doctor if you experience symptoms of Vitamin A deficiency. Your doctor will conclude by examining your history and physical examination and may ask for a serum retinol test if necessary.

Vitamin A Diagnostic Test

A serum retinol blood test is used to measure the amount of Vitamin A in your blood.

A blood sample is taken from your vein on an empty stomach. Alcohol should not be consumed for 24 hours before sample collection.

The healthy range for adults is 20 to 80 mcg/dL. If your reading is less than 20 mcg/dL, you are Vitamin A deficient. However, this test is not accurate because your body stores large amounts of Vitamin A in the liver, so your blood Vitamin A levels will not decrease until your liver stores of Vitamin A are depleted.

The gold standard to assess the overall Vitamin A levels in the body is by measuring the concentration of retinol in the liver through a biopsy. Liver biopsies pose significant risks, so they are not commonly used to assess Vitamin A levels.

If you have a Vitamin A deficiency, your healthcare provider may prescribe high doses of a Vitamin A supplement for a few days. Once your symptoms begin to improve, they will likely switch you to a lower dose of Vitamin A.

If your retinol level is above 30 mcg/dL, taking Vitamin A supplements may not be helpful and may even cause toxicity. In this case, it's better to focus on consuming foods that are naturally rich in Vitamin A.

What am I missing if I'm not consuming enough Vitamin A?

Let us look at the important functions and health benefits of Vitamin A in detail in the next chapter.

CHAPTER 2

IMPORTANCE OF VITAMIN A

Vitamin A is involved in various physiological processes of the body. It plays various important roles through which it maintains the body's functions and prevents various diseases. First, let's see its important roles in the body.

Is Vitamin A an antioxidant?

Yes and no!

Yes, because Vitamin A enhances the antioxidant response of the body. And no, because Vitamin A is not directly involved in killing free radicals like true antioxidants. Instead, it regulates genes that help the body respond to and prevent oxidative stress. This is why Vitamin A can't technically be classified as a true antioxidant, it's more like an indirect antioxidant. While Vitamin A isn't technically a true antioxidant, it plays an important role in strengthening the body's antioxidant capacity and preventing the formation of harmful free radicals that can damage DNA. This can ultimately help prevent the onset of chronic diseases like diabetes, heart disease, cancer, respiratory issues, autoimmune disorders, infectious diseases, and neurological conditions.

Are carotenoids antioxidants?

Yes, carotenoids are true antioxidants. There are more than 500 different carotenoids, and most of them, including provitamin A carotenoids - beta-carotene, alpha-carotene, and beta-cryptoxanthin, are known for their antioxidant activity.

Carotenoids are very potent natural antioxidants. These carotenoids are highly effective at quenching singlet oxygen and scavenging reactive oxygen species found in cellular lipid bilayers. Beta-carotene, for instance, targets lipophilic radicals within each cell compartment and chelates oxygen-free radicals and eliminates their energy, thus avoiding peroxidation of lipids and guarding against damage caused by free radicals.

Due to their antioxidant properties, carotenoids can help reduce or even prevent the development of various free radical-related disorders, such as autoimmune diseases, cognitive disorders, diabetes, heart disease, and different types of cancer.

ROLE OF VITAMIN A IN THE BODY

The Important Anti-inflammatory Action of Vitamin A

Insufficient Vitamin A intake can cause inflammation and worsen existing inflammatory conditions. This deficiency may also contribute to the onset of Alzheimer's disease. In addition, persistent inflammation can lead to chronic ailments, including diabetes, heart disease, rheumatoid arthritis, cancer, and psoriasis.

Vitamin A is beneficial in various inflammatory issues, such as acne, Alzheimer's disease, bronchopulmonary dysplasia, and certain precancerous and cancerous states. This vitamin is regarded as an anti-inflammatory agent due to its vital role in strengthening the immune system. It helps regulate the immune system's response and prevent overreaction that may cause inflammation.

Vitamin A exists in three forms: retinol, retinal, and retinoic acid (RA), with the latter having the most biological activity. RA converts into two crucial derivatives, namely, 9-cis-retinoic acid and all-trans-retinoic acid (ATRA). Retinoid acids play a role in regulating the differentiation, maturation, and function of innate immune system cells, which is composed of macrophages and neutrophil. These cells respond immediately to pathogen invasion by activating natural killer T cells that carry out important immune regulatory functions. Macrophages include M1 macrophages that release pro-inflammatory cytokines and M2 macrophages that express anti-inflammatory factors. All-trans-retinoic acid (ATRA), a derivative of retinoid acid, can inhibit inflammatory responses by preventing macrophages from releasing inflammatory factors and inducing the conversion of M1 to M2 macrophages in the bone marrow.

Recent research has found that beta-carotene can help slow down the progression of rheumatoid arthritis. This is because beta-carotene inhibits the translocation of nuclear factor kappa B, reducing the transcription of pro-inflammatory cytokine genes such as interleukins and tumor necrosis factor-alpha (TNF-α). Beta-carotene is further converted into Vitamin A in the body, which is then metabolized into all-trans-retinoic acid (ATRA), which has anti-inflammatory properties. Consuming fruits and vegetables that are high in beta-carotene can have these positive effects, while supplements have been found to be ineffective.

What are the active forms of Vitamin A?

After you eat food, your body metabolizes Vitamin A and provitamin A into biologically active forms: retinol, retinal, and retinoic acid. Vitamin A exerts all of its action through these biologically active forms. All these three forms are toxic at high levels. Vitamin A levels can easily reach toxic levels when excessive Vitamin A supplements are taken. This is the reason why it is recommended to get Vitamin A from green and yellow vegetables, fruits, and dairy products rather than through dietary supplements.

Why is Vitamin A important?

1. Eyesight

Maintaining eye health is the most important and well-known function of Vitamin A. Having normal levels of Vitamin A is crucial for good vision, as having too much or too little can be harmful. Vitamin A plays a major role in the visual cycle and color vision, and its deficiency can cause vision loss and blindness.

Vitamin A is a component of the protein rhodopsin, a highly sensitive to the light pigment found in the retina within the eye. It allows the eyes to see in low-light environments, basically helping you see better in the dark. Vitamin A not only supports the vision function but also maintains the covering and lining of the eyes. It supports normal differentiation and function of the conjunctival membranes and cornea.

Another essential function of Vitamin A is that it is involved in visual phototransduction, which is the process that converts light into electrical signals. These signals from the retina travel through the optic nerve to the brain and are converted into an image.

Difficulty seeing in dim light is a characteristic of night blindness. It is an early sign of Vitamin A deficiency. If there are insufficient rhodopsin levels, the retina struggles to convert provitamin A carotenoids into Vitamin A, leading to temporary blindness in dark spots.

Inadequate intake of Vitamin A in the diet can gradually lead to complete vision loss over time. Vitamin A deficiency can cause dysfunction of the lining and covering of the eyes, leading to xerophthalmia or dry eyes. This condition can progress and even result in ulcers in the cornea, eventually causing blindness.

2. Skin Integrity

Vitamin A plays a vital role in maintaining the integrity and function of the skin. Vitamin A helps in the daily replacement of skin cells. Melanogenesis is the process by which melanocytes produce the pigment melanin, which provides skin color and protects deeper skin layers from the sun's DNA-damaging ultraviolet radiation. The phototransduction cascade, which initiates melanogenesis, requires Retinal (the active form of Vitamin A). In addition, retinoic acid regulates the melanocyte stem cells and influences melanocyte differentiation and proliferation. Vitamin A plays a crucial role in maintaining the integrity and function of the skin. Vitamin A helps in the daily replacement of skin cells. Melanogenesis is the process by which melanocytes produce the pigment melanin, which provides skin color and protects deeper skin layers from the sun's DNA-damaging ultraviolet radiation. The phototransduction cascade, which initiates melanogenesis, requires Retinal (the active form of Vitamin A). In addition, retinoic acid regulates the melanocyte stem cells and influences melanocyte differentiation and proliferation.

3. Hair Health

Vitamin A is an important micronutrient for hair growth. Vitamin A is essential for cell growth, which, in turn, helps your hair grow, but both too little and too much Vitamin A can have harmful effects. Retinoic acid, which is the biologically active form of Vitamin A, plays a significant role in regulating hair follicle stem cells and affecting the hair cycle's functioning. Additionally, Vitamin A aids in sebum production, which is a natural oil produced by skin glands on the scalp. Sebum helps hydrate the scalp, reduces frizz, and prevents breakage, ultimately promoting healthy hair growth.

4. Reproduction and Embryogenesis

Vitamin A metabolite, known as all-trans retinoic acid, plays a vital role in male and female reproductive systems, as well as in various events during the development of an embryo.

Moreover, Vitamin A is crucial for the upkeep of the male genital tract, aiding in the growth of sperm. Recent studies suggest that Vitamin A also supports the developing tissues of a fetus in the womb and aids in the formation of the placenta during pregnancy.

5. Cell Growth

Vitamin A is crucial in regulating the growth and differentiation of many types of cells. All cells are derived from stem cells and acquire their functions as they mature. Cell differentiation is the process by which cells acquire distinct roles as they divide. Vitamin A plays a role in cell proliferation, differentiation, and function by impacting the biosynthesis of various proteins, including those that regulate growth and cell function. Additionally, Vitamin A is involved in determining a cell's sensitivity to hormones and hormone-like factors. Studies suggest that Vitamin A also influences the production of secretory proteins that act as hormones.

6. Development Process (Central Nervous System)

Vitamin A is crucial for early development and signaling functions in the human brain and requires a delicate balance for optimal functioning. Retinoids, which are Vitamin A derivatives found in the central nervous system, regulate neuronal differentiation and neural tube patterning - the process by which cells in the developing nervous system gain specific identities.

Vitamin A plays a significant role in maintaining high function in the central nervous system and is essential for both the development and operation of the olfactory system. Retinoic acid, a Vitamin A metabolite, is involved in olfaction (sense of smell) and cognitive activities such as memory, learning, and spatial functions.

Studies have found lower levels of Vitamin A and beta-carotene in Alzheimer's disease (AD) patients. The degradation of retinoic acid signaling may influence the initiation and development of Alzheimer's disease. More importantly, research has shown that Vitamin A can slow the progression of Alzheimer's disease. Vitamin A has also been shown to protect against other brain diseases such as Parkinson's disease, cerebral ischemia, autism, and schizophrenia.

7. Bone Health

It was previously believed that Vitamin A increases bone resorption (breaking down of old bones) and prevents the building of new bones. If you take too much Vitamin A (more than 3,000 mcg or 10,000 IU/day), it can even increase the risk of fractures. However, recent studies have shown that not having enough Vitamin A can also increase the risk of fractures. More research has shown that Vitamin A (in the right amounts) can actually help promote healthy bones. Additionally, provitamin A (carotene and beta-cryptoxanthin) may also protect bones.

Carotene and beta-cryptoxanthin help with bone formation and can prevent the activation of nuclear factor-kappa B to inhibit the differentiation as well as maturation of osteoclasts (cells that break down bone). Both Vitamin A and provitamin A are important for building strong, healthy bones and can potentially prevent bone fractures.

8. Immunity

Vitamin A plays a vital role in immune system regulation. It protects against various infections and inflammatory and allergic diseases. Vitamin A deficiency increases your susceptibility to infection. All-trans-retinoic acid is the active form of Vitamin A, which has anti-inflammatory properties and is essential for generating both innate and adaptive immune cell responses. Vitamin A has an impact on the activation of neutrophils and macrophages. Additionally, it plays a significant role in regulating the differentiation of T-helper cells and B cells. In addition, Vitamin A has an important role in mucus secretion, providing the first line of defense against foreign bodies entering the body. Vitamin A provides mechanistic protection by playing an essential role in the formation and function of epithelial cells.

9. Red Blood Cell Formation

Retinoic acid, which is the active component of Vitamin A, regulates the hormone erythropoietin for a short period. Erythropoietin stimulates red blood cell production. Retinoids potentially control the programmed cell death of red blood cell precursors. Moreover, Vitamin A has the ability to enhance the mobility of iron from the liver to developing red blood cells, which helps in the incorporation of iron into hemoglobin. Hemoglobin is responsible for carrying oxygen in red blood cells.

10. Thyroid Function

Vitamin A reduces the risk of hypothyroidism. Vitamin A deficiency negatively impacts the thyroid health. Not enough Vitamin A in the body can cause the pituitary gland to create and release more thyroid-stimulating hormone (TSH). This can result in the thyroid gland becoming larger and less able to uptake iodine. Vitamin A activates thyroid hormone receptors, regulates thyroid hormone metabolism, and inhibits thyroid-stimulating hormone (TSH) secretion, thereby reducing the risk of goiter.

IN DISEASE PREVENTION AND TREATMENTS

As Vitamin A plays an important part in various physiological functions of the body, having enough Vitamin A can prevent and effectively be used in various disease treatments. Especially beta carotene from plant sources has more advanced protective effects than preformed Vitamin A. Let's see how Vitamin A is significant in different disease prevention and control:

1. Prevent Cancer

Vitamin A from plant sources is more effective in protecting against cancer than supplements. Some clinical trial suggests that Vitamin A supplements may reduce the risk of some cancers but at the same time increase the risk of other forms of cancer, such as prostate cancer, cardiovascular disease morbidity, and mortality. High-dose supplements of carotenoids may increase the risk of lung cancer in smokers.

Consuming a diet that is abundant in micronutrients, particularly Vitamin A, can boost the immune system and prognosis for individuals with head and neck cancer. It may also decrease the likelihood of developing oral and pharyngeal cancer.

Studies have suggested that Vitamin A and carotenoids have protective potential against the development of breast cancer. Vitamin A and carotenoids are potent antioxidants and are highly effective at scavenging free radicals, which helps to protect against photooxidative damage. They also protect breast cancer development and progression by inhibiting cell proliferation, survival, and invasion.

2. Acute Promyelocytic Leukemia

Myeloid stem cells in the bone marrow normally differentiate into platelets, red blood cells, and white blood cells (also known as leukocytes), which are crucial for the immune response. However, if myeloid cell differentiation is disrupted, it can lead to the overgrowth of immature white blood cells, causing leukemia. In people with Acute promyelocytic leukemia, administering high doses of all-trans retinoic acid (ATRA), an active metabolite of Vitamin A, can help restore normal differentiation and greatly improve chances of complete remission.

3. Measles

Measles is a viral infection that attacks the respiratory system and may spread to other parts of the body. It poses a serious threat to young children. One of the major risk factors for severe measles is a lack of Vitamin A. Consuming enough Vitamin A can help prevent measles and reduce mortality rates for those who contract the infection. World Health Organization recommends higher doses of Vitamin A to children over six months old who are malnourished, immunocompromised, or at risk of complications from measles.

4. Age-Related Macular Degeneration

Age-related macular degeneration (AMD) is an eye disease that can make your central vision blurry. The macula, which is responsible for sharp and direct vision and is a part of the retina (the tissue that is sensitive to light and located at the back of the eye), becomes damaged as you age. This condition is called age-related macular degeneration. As people get older, their risk of developing age-related macular degeneration increases, which is the most common cause of blindness in elderly people. This disease is complex and caused by genetic and environmental factors, such as aging, smoking, obesity, and high oxidative stress.

Vitamin A is an essential nutrient for the human eye and plays an important role in human retinal pigment epithelial cells. Several studies suggest a positive association between a reduction in dietary micronutrient intake and the progression of age-related macular degeneration. Micronutrients with antioxidant capacity may prevent oxidative stress involved in the development of degenerative eye diseases. The risk of macular degeneration can be effectively reduced by consuming foods rich in antioxidants such as beta-carotene, which has a protective effect on age-related macular degeneration. Long-term consumption of fruits and vegetables containing provitamin A carotenoid reduces the risk of any stage of AMD.

5. Prevention of Heart Disease

Cardiovascular disease (CVD) is a major cause of death worldwide, and its prevention is crucial. Vitamins, especially those with antioxidant properties, can play an essential role in preventing and treating cardiovascular disease. Vitamin A and provitamin A carotenoids can reduce oxidative stress by acting as antioxidants. The development of cardiovascular diseases is believed to be significantly influenced by oxidative stress.

Vitamin A and carotenoids possess anti-inflammatory and antioxidant properties, making them important for reducing the incidence of heart disease. These compounds are effective in mitigating and protecting against various forms of cardiovascular diseases, such as atherosclerosis, hypertension, arrhythmias, myocardial ischemia, and heart failure. Research indicates that high levels of Vitamin A in the body can reduce both systolic and diastolic blood pressure in individuals with hypertension.

Vitamin A can reduce atherosclerosis due to its antioxidant and anti-inflammatory properties. Reports indicate that Vitamin A can lower oxidative stress levels in diabetic patients with ischemic heart disease. Additionally, beta-carotene can reduce the size of ischemia-reperfusion-induced infarcts and improve post-ischemic cardiac function recovery.

Eating red, green, and orange vegetables and fruits can provide the heart-protective effects associated with Vitamin A. While taking vitamin supplements may not provide many cardiovascular benefits, getting Vitamin A and beta carotene from food is recommended.

6. Treating Skin Disorders

Vitamin A is used topically and taken orally to treat various skin conditions. From severe acne to premature aging, warts, and psoriasis, Vitamin A and its derivatives can work wonders for your skin.

In fact, Vitamin A was the first Vitamin Approved by the Food and Drug Administration as an anti-wrinkle agent. It can change the appearance of your skin surface and has anti-aging effects. Retinoids, which are derivatives of Vitamin A, play a crucial role in cell division, differentiation, and cell death. They can promote keratinocyte proliferation, which are skin cells that secrete keratin - a protein that protects against microbial invasion, shields against U.V. exposure, and maintains skin hydration.

Vitamin A strengthens the protective function of your skin, limits transepidermal water loss, and protects collagen against degradation. It's also been shown to have beneficial effects on skin diseases with disturbances of keratinization, such as psoriasis. In psoriasis, skin cells build up, forming scales and itchy and dry patches. Vitamin A can help improve psoriasis symptoms by reducing the formation of inflammation-causing proteins, cytokines, and interleukins.

7. Wound Healing

The growth and differentiation of various cell types within the skin are regulated by Vitamin A. It plays a crucial role in the inflammatory phase of wound healing. In damaged tissue, Vitamin A promotes the renewal of skin cells, accelerates the process of tissue regeneration, and helps in maintaining the structure of the epithelial layer. The process of epithelialization involves the migration of epithelial cells upwards to repair the wounded area. This process is vital to wound healing. Also, Vitamin A can reverse the inhibitory effects of anti-inflammatory steroids on wound healing. Vitamin A enhances the production of collagen type I and fibronectin, which are essential for tissue repair. It also increases the proliferation of keratinocytes, which are required to restore the epidermal barrier and fibroblasts, which are necessary for reducing the size of the wound.

8. Sunburn

Skin exposure to sunlight is crucial for the production of Vitamin D, but long-term exposure to UV-A radiation (315-400 nm) can penetrate deep layers of the skin epidermis and generate free radicals that lead to premature skin aging. Both Vitamin A and provitamin A carotenoids protect against the harmful effects of sunlight. Carotenoids, especially beta-carotene and canthaxanthin, act as protective agents for the skin by scavenging free radicals.

Your body stores Vitamin A in the form of retinyl esters, which are concentrated in the skin and can absorb ultraviolet radiation. Applying retinyl palmitate (a form of Vitamin A) topically is as effective as using a sunscreen with a sun protection factor 20 in preventing sunburn erythema and the formation of thymine dimers, which can cause DNA damage in the skin and ultimately lead to skin cancer.

CHAPTER 3

10 BEST FOODS RICH IN VITAMIN A

The shortcut rule to identify food rich in Vitamin A is RYG, i.e., Red, Yellow, and Green. Red, yellow, and green colored fruits and vegetables are good sources of vitamin A. Here are the top 10 foods that are high in Vitamin A.

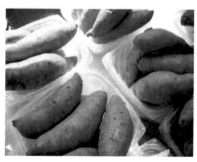

1. Sweet Potato

All varieties of sweet potatoes, orange, white, and purple, are good sources of vitamin A, but sweet potatoes with orange-yellow flesh are an excellent source of vitamin A because they have the highest levels of beta-carotene. One whole cooked orange sweet potato with the skin on provides 156% of the daily requirement for vitamin A. The deeper the orange color of the sweet potato, the more beta-carotene it contains. Beta carotene converts into vitamin A in the body and effectively reduces the risk of developing prostate cancer and colorectal cancer.

Purple fleshed sweet potatoes are low in beta-carotene and high in anthocyanin. This potent antioxidant may help reduce inflammation, improve neurological health, and protect against various non-communicable diseases.

Sweet potatoes are high in vitamin A as well as vitamin C, both of which are potent antioxidants that boost your immune system and protect against infection. The high fiber content of sweet potatoes promotes proper digestion and prevents constipation.

2. Spinach

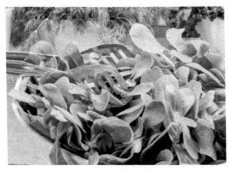

Spinach is a superfood because it is rich in many nutrients. Spinach is one of the best sources of Vitamin A. Half a cup of boiled spinach fulfills 64% of your daily vitamin A requirement. It not only improves vision and boosts your immune system but also prevents diabetes and high blood pressure. This leafy vegetable is also an excellent source of iron, calcium, and vitamin K. This means that by eating spinach regularly, you get strong bones and have thick hair and glowing skin. Spinach contains oxalates, which reduce the absorption of important nutrients of spinach in the body. To reduce the oxalate content of spinach, blanch it in enough water to reduce oxalate by 30%-87% and increase your body's absorption of nutrients.

3. Carrots

Carrots are rich in carotenoid antioxidants, especially beta-carotene. One cup or 100 grams of raw carrots fulfills 104% of your daily requirement of Vitamin A and keeps your eyes healthy. In addition to beta-carotene, carrots

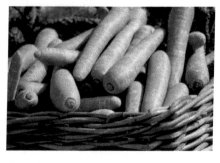

contain alpha-carotene that is partially metabolized into vitamin A in the body, as well as other potent antioxidants such as gamma-carotene, lutein (mostly in orange carrots), lycopene (mostly in red carrots), and zeaxanthin that reduce the risk of cancer and heart disease. Their soluble fiber content is high, which lowers cholesterol levels by binding to cholesterol particles and carrying them out of the body.

4. Pumpkin

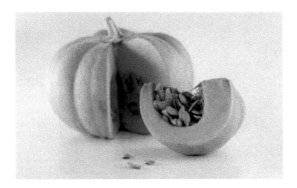

Pumpkin is an excellent source of beta-carotene. 100 grams of raw pumpkin fulfills 53% of your daily requirement of Vitamin A. Being high in beta-carotene, which eventually converts into vitamin A in the body, pumpkin lowers the risk of cataracts, strengthens your immune system, and provides protection against asthma. Along with vitamin A, pumpkin is also a good source of lutein and zeaxanthin. These two antioxidants fight free radicals in the body and reduce the risk of age-related macular degeneration. Pumpkin contains very few calories, which makes it weight-friendly. Instead of buying canned pumpkin purée, make the purée at home to avoid consuming excessive sugar and preservatives. You can make pumpkin pudding and pumpkin cake or use pumpkin purée as a pasta sauce.

> ***Read 10 Smart Ways to Incorporate Pumpkin into Your Diet in Eat So What! Smart Ways to Stay Healthy.***

5. Kale

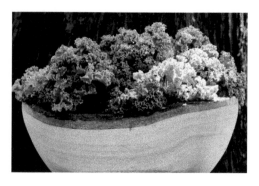

Kale is one of the healthiest vegetables. It is rich in many vitamins and minerals and is low in calories. 100 grams of raw kale contains 35% of the daily recommended value of vitamin A. Cooking reduces the vitamin A content of kale by up to 20%, so eat them raw to get the most vitamin A. Kale is also a good source of Vitamin C and K. Powerful antioxidants like quercetin and kaempferol present in kale help reduce the risk of cancer and heart disease.

If you have thyroid or kidney problems or are taking blood thinners, consult your doctor before including them in your diet. Consuming kale in excess hinders the functioning of the thyroid. Vitamin K plays a vital role in the process of blood clotting and interferes with blood-thinning medicines' activity. People with kidney problems should limit their intake of high-potassium vegetables like kale.

6. Muskmelon/ Cantaloupe Melon

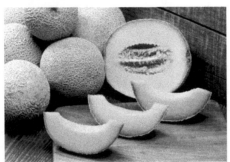

Cantaloupe is quite an underrated fruit. It is rich in beta carotene as well as vitamin C. 100 grams of raw cantaloupe provides 21% of the day's requirement of Vitamin A and 44% of Vitamin C. The best thing about cantaloupe is that it is mostly water and has zero fat and cholesterol. It also prevents and controls diabetes as well as high blood pressure. Watermelon is low in carbs and has a low glycemic index. It slowly releases glucose into the blood and does not allow blood sugar to rise, which makes it a diabetic-friendly fruit. Potassium-rich cantaloupe keeps your blood pressure under control and keeps your heart healthy. The high fiber and water content present in cantaloupe keeps your digestion healthy. Before cutting the melon, wash it thoroughly under running water and scrub the outer surface to remove any bacteria that may be present. Melons are known to be susceptible to contamination, so taking this precaution is important.

7. Red Bell Pepper

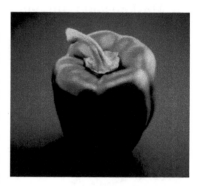

Red bell peppers is a great source of Vitamin A. Among green, yellow, and red bell peppers, bell peppers contain the most beta-carotene, which is converted into vitamin A in the body. 100 grams of red bell pepper fulfills 21% of the daily vitamin A requirement, almost 10 times more than green bell peppers. The red bell pepper is the fully ripened variety and the most nutritious of the three types. They are also a good vitamin C, potassium, magnesium, calcium, and iron source. Due to the high vitamin C content, red bell peppers help prevent anemia by increasing iron absorption in the body. However, the heat dilutes some of the health benefits of bell peppers, so eating it raw in a salad will give you maximum health benefits.

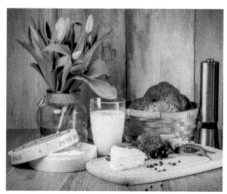

8. Cheese

Although cheese isn't the healthiest source of vitamin A, at least you can eat cheese a little guilt-free. Unlike sugar, cheese isn't solely about calories, it also provides some nutrition. Ricotta cheese and cheddar cheese are good sources of vitamin A. 100 grams of Cheddar and Ricotta cheese provide 45% and 18% of Vitamin A, respectively. This means 1 slice (17 grams) of cheddar and ricotta cheese provides 8% and 3% of vitamin A, respectively. Make sure you choose healthier varieties of cheese like cottage, ricotta, and cheddar instead of processed cheese. Avoid processed cheese completely as this variety has high calories and negligible health benefits, and it increases the cholesterol level in the body.

9. Mango

The summer season is incomplete without mangoes. They are not only delicious but also fulfill your daily

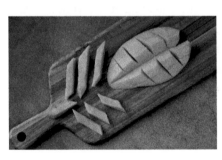

requirement of Vitamin A. One whole mango contains 12% of the daily value of vitamin A. The high-water content and fiber in mangoes help in reducing constipation. A mango a day can stabilize your digestive system and help keep bowel movements normal. This sweet juicy fruit keeps your eyes healthy and boosts your immunity. Mango makes your bones strong and keeps your reproductive system healthy. Apart from vitamin A, mangoes are rich in vitamin C and folate.

10. Papaya

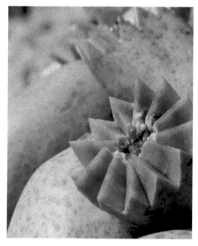

100 grams of papaya contains 9% of a day's recommended intake of vitamin A. Papaya is also an excellent Vitamin C source. 100 grams of papaya fulfills 75% of the Vitamin C requirement of the day. Papaya is low in calories, and about 88% of it consists of water, making it a favorable fruit for weight loss. Antioxidants like Vitamin A and C in papaya boost immunity, fight free radicals, and reduce inflammation in the body, thus preventing chronic diseases like heart disease and cancer. The high fiber content of papaya improves digestion by relieving constipation.

CHAPTER 4

POTENTIALLY DANGEROUS VITAMIN A COMBINATIONS YOU SHOULD AVOID

VITAMIN A + VITAMIN K

Consuming excessive amounts of Vitamin A can hinder Vitamin K absorption in the body, which is necessary for effective blood clotting. However, consuming vitamin A-rich foods in moderation is unlikely to have a significant impact on Vitamin K absorption, but taking high doses of Vitamin A supplements may significantly decrease the effectiveness of vitamin K.

VITAMIN A + BLOOD THINNERS

If you are taking an anticoagulant or blood-thinning medication, such as warfarin, limiting your consumption of foods rich in Vitamin A is important. This is because taking Vitamin A with blood-thinning medication may increase the risk of bleeding events, which can be particularly dangerous if you are also taking vitamin A supplements. However, some studies suggest that Vitamin A supplements can be safely taken by individuals who require chronic warfarin therapy. It is recommended to maintain a 2-hour gap between taking warfarin and Vitamin A supplements. Alternatively, you should consult your doctor and pharmacist regarding your supplement and food consumption while taking blood-thinning medication.

VITAMIN A + WATER-SOLUBLE VITAMINS

In order to receive the health benefits of vitamins, they must be properly absorbed. It's not recommended to take fat-soluble vitamin A with water-soluble vitamins (B complex and C) because they are absorbed differently in the body. Combining them may reduce the health benefits you receive from each. Water-soluble vitamins are well absorbed on an empty stomach, while fat-soluble vitamins require the presence of fat in the body to be adequately absorbed. To maximize the benefits of each type of vitamin, consume B and C-rich foods in the morning and foods rich in vitamin A in the evening. If you take vitamin supplements, take B and C on an empty stomach and take vitamin A in the evening after a meal.

CHAPTER 5

VITAMIN A COMBINATIONS FOR SYNERGISTIC HEALTH BENEFITS

VITAMIN A + IRON

A lack of Vitamin A can have an impact on iron metabolism, which can lead to anemia. Although

Vitamin A deficiency does not decrease iron absorption, it can reduce the synthesis of hemoglobin. To combat anemia, it is recommended to consume foods that are high in both iron and vitamin A. Studies have shown that combining vitamin A with iron is more effective in increasing hemoglobin levels than consuming iron alone. This is because Vitamin A enhances iron utilization in the body.

Let's understand the science behind it:

Seeds, legumes, and grains like wheat, rice, and corn (yes, corn kernels are considered grains!) contain phytic acid, which is an anti-nutrient. Phytic acid binds with minerals like iron, zinc, calcium, and magnesium in the body, creating phytates that prevent the minerals from being absorbed properly. Without absorption, you can't reap the full benefits of these minerals.

These phytates can only be broken down by an enzyme called phytase, which releases the minerals and makes them available for absorption in the body. The problem is that there's very little phytase in the small intestine, which hinders the body's ability to digest phytates. This means that even if you're consuming enough minerals like iron, you may not be getting their full benefits. Interestingly, even though phytate may hinder mineral absorption, having undigested phytate in the colon may actually protect against colonic carcinoma.

Vitamin A (and beta-carotene, which converts to vitamin A in the body) can counteract the inhibitory effect of phytates on iron absorption. Vitamin A forms a complex with iron, which remains soluble in the intestine even at a pH of 6. This increases the availability of iron in the bloodstream for absorption.

Research indicates that normal levels of vitamin A (up to 900 µg) favor iron absorption. However, high doses of vitamin A (1800 µg) may lower iron absorption in the body. These high doses of vitamin A are generally possible with vitamin A supplements, not with foods. For best results, get these nutrients from natural food sources, not from vitamin supplements. Eat foods high in vitamin A, such as sweet potatoes, carrots, and pumpkin, with iron food sources such as beans, lentils, and spinach for maximum health benefits.

VITAMIN A + ZINC

Not having enough zinc in your diet can lead to a deficiency in vitamin A. To ensure you get the maximum health benefits of vitamin A, it's important to eat it with zinc-rich food sources. Zinc is crucial for all aspects of vitamin A metabolism, including absorption, transport, and utilization in the body. Without enough zinc, vitamin A (1) cannot be absorbed in the intestine (2) cannot be converted into retinal, therefore cannot be then converted to its active form (3) cannot be transported from blood circulation to body tissues, (4) cannot be released from its storage form, in the liver when needed. This limits the body's ability to use the vitamin A you consume. The combination of vitamin A and zinc also positively impacts your immunity, with vitamin A playing an important role in the production and function of white blood cells, and zinc is required for the development and function of cell-mediating innate immunity, natural killer cells, and neutrophils. Both nutrients also have antioxidant properties and help fight free radicals in the body. By eating them together, you can protect yourself against numerous chronic diseases.

To maximize the health benefits of vitamin A, eat foods rich in this nutrient, such as spinach, sweet potatoes, and red bell peppers, alongside zinc-rich options like chickpeas, kidney beans, cashews, pumpkin seeds, and oats.

CHAPTER 6

DIET PLAN

Here's a 10-day diet plan to include natural sources rich in vitamin A in your diet. Repeat this diet plan every 10 days and you will never be deficient in vitamin A.

Day 1: 1 baked sweet potato with skin (>100%).

Day 2: ⅔ cup ice cream (20%) + 1 large cooked red bell pepper (15%) + 1 cup carrot juice (>65%).

Day 3: 2 slices of papaya (20%) + ½ cup raw carrots (50%) + 1 cup vanilla ice-cream (30%).

Day 4: 1 piece of pumpkin pie (55%) + 2 slices of cantaloupe (25%)+ 2 mangoes (20%).

Day 5: ½ cup cooked spinach* (65%) + ½ cup raw carrots (50%).

Day 6: 100 g cooked kale (55%) + 2 large mangoes (30%) + 30 g cheddar cheese (15%).

Day 7: 1 baked sweet potato with skin (>100%).

Day 8: ½ cup ricotta cheese (15%) + 1 cup milk (20%) + ½ cup cooked spinach (65%).

Day 9: 100 g pumpkin (55%) + 2 slices of papaya (20%) + 1½ cup milk shake (25%).

Day 10: 100 g pumpkin (55%) + 2 slices of cantaloupe (25%) +1 cup milk (20%).

CHAPTER 7

RECIPES

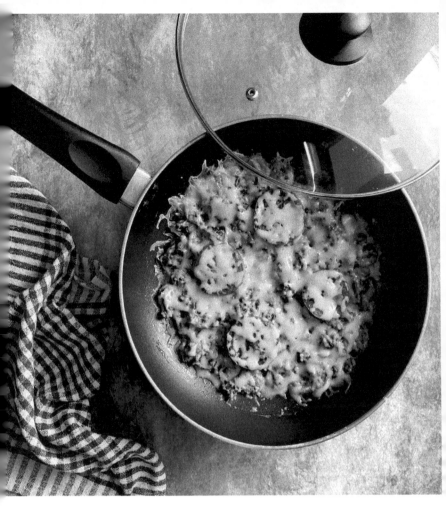

Pan Fried Cheesy Mushrooms

Ingredients

Button mushroom: 200 g	Cheddar cheese: 50 g
Cashew nuts: 30	Garlic: 5

Tomato: 1	Black pepper powder: ¼ tsp
Salt: To taste	Water: 100 ml
Butter: 1 tbsp	

Method

1. Wash and chop the mushrooms. Soak cashews in hot water for 2 hours. Grind them with water to make a thick paste.

2. Heat butter in a pan. Add chopped garlic to it and cook till it turns crisp. Take out the garlic from the pan.

3. Add chopped mushrooms, salt and black pepper powder. Cover and cook till all the water released by the mushrooms is re-absorbed.

4. Add cashew paste and mix well so that all the mushrooms get coated well in the paste. Cover with the lid and cook for 10 minutes. If it is sticking, then add 2 tbsp water.

5. Place tomato slices on top. Sprinkle salt and black pepper powder on the tomato slices. Cover and cook for 5 minutes till the tomatoes become soft.

6. Sprinkle fried garlic and shredded cheddar cheese over the mushrooms. Keep it covered for 2 minutes till the cheese melts.

7. Turn off the flame and enjoy piping hot Pan-Fried Cheesy Mushrooms.

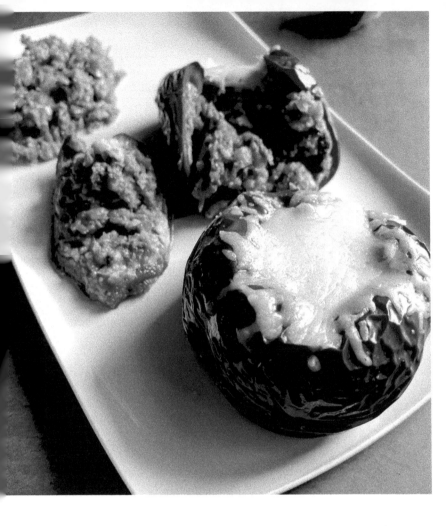

Stuffed Bell Pepper

Ingredients

Red bell pepper: 4	Cottage cheese: 200 g
Cheddar cheese: 100 g	Chopped garlic: 2 tbsp
Chopped onion: 50 g	Chopped carrot: 50 g
Chopped cabbage: 50 g	Chopped tomato: 50 g

Chopped pumpkin: 50 g	Chopped green bell pepper: 50 g
Chopped mushroom: 50 g	Mixed herbs (oregano, parsley, thyme): 1 tbsp
Red chili pepper: ½ tsp	Salt: To taste
Oil: 2 tbsp	

Method

1. Preheat the oven to 190 °C.

2. Heat oil in a pan. Add chopped garlic and cook for 2 minutes. Add onion and cook for 5 minutes.

3. Add all the chopped vegetables one by one and cook until mushrooms and tomato release water.

4. Add salt, red chili pepper, mixed herbs (or your choice of herbs) and mix well.

5. Lastly, add crumbled cottage cheese and cook the stuffing until it becomes slightly dry. Turn off the flame.

6. Remove the tops of the peppers and scoop out the seeds. Grease the outer side of the pepper with oil and sprinkle some salt.

7. Grate some cheese inside the pepper and fill it with the prepared stuffing. Press the stuffing with the fingertip.

8. Place the bell peppers upside down in a baking tray and bake for 25 minutes at 190°C.

9. Remove the peppers and sprinkle a generous amount of cheese on top. Bake again, keeping the cheese side on top for 5 minutes until the cheese is melted.

Sarso ka Saag

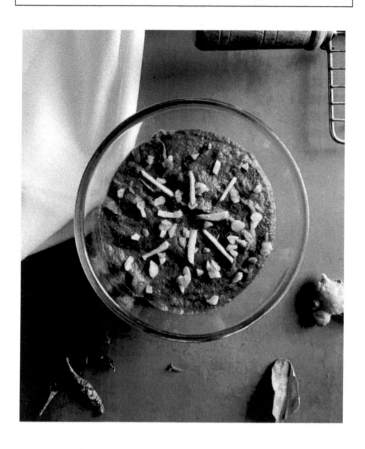

Ingredients

Mustard greens: 175 g
Spinach: 75 g
Lemon juice: 1 tbsp
Maize flour: 2 tbsp
Asafoetida: ¼ tsp
Cumin seeds: ½ tsp
Ginger: 1 inch
Garlic: 5 cloves
Onion: 3
Tomato: 1 medium
Garam masala: 1 tsp
Coriander powder: 1 tsp

Salt: To taste   Water: 250 ml
Rice bran oil: 2 tbsp

For Tampering

Ginger julienne: 1 tbsp   Chopped garlic: 1 tbsp
Asafoetida: A pinch   Red chilli: 1
Butter: 1 tsp

Method

1. Wash the mustard greens and spinach thoroughly. Cut them roughly.

2. Blanch the greens with 50 ml water, salt, and lemon juice for 5 minutes or till the greens are soft.

3. Let it cool down completely. Make a thick puree by grinding the greens with stock and green chilies.

4. Heat oil in a pan. Add asafoetida and cumin. Cook for one minute.

5. Add chopped ginger and garlic. Cook for 2-3 minutes.

6. Add chopped onions. Cover with a lid and cook on low flame for 10 minutes.

7. Add chopped tomatoes and salt (we have added salt during blanching, so add salt accordingly). Cover with a lid and cook on low flame for 10 minutes. Mash the tomatoes with a spatula.

8. Add garam masala and coriander powder. Mix well and cook for 5 minutes.

9. Add maize flour and mix well. Cook for 2 minutes. Add mustard greens and spinach puree and mix well.

10. Add 200 ml water and cook on low flame for 10 minutes. Keep stirring in between, and do not cover the greens. Turn off the flame and add tempering.

For Tempering

1. Heat butter in a pan and add asafoetida, ginger, garlic, and red chili to it. Cook the garlic till it turns brown.

2. Add this tempering to the prepared mustard greens. Immediately cover the greens with a lid. Keep aside for 10 minutes.

3. Enjoy Sarson ka Saag with makki ki roti (maize flour flatbread).

Tips:

1. You can also add other greens like chenopodium, collard, and radish greens with spinach. If using mixed greens, add 125 grams of mustard greens and 125 grams of mixed greens.

2. To retain the bright green color of the greens, do not cover them while blanching.

4. Very little salt is needed in sarson ka saag. You may need half or a quarter of the normal amount. So, add salt according to your taste.

The End

Sign up to La Fonceur Newsletter to receive Bonus Recipes:

https://eatsowhat.com/signup

READ THE EAT SO WHAT! SERIES

Book 1

Eat So What! Smart Ways to Stay Healthy

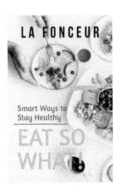

Book 2

Eat So What! The Power of Vegetarianism

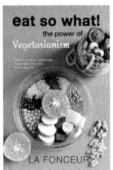

REFERENCES

1. Albahrani AA, Greaves RF. Fat-Soluble Vitamins: Clinical Indications and Current Challenges for Chromatographic Measurement. Clin Biochem Rev. 2016 Feb;37(1):27-46.

2. Multivitamin/Mineral Supplements Fact Sheet for Health Professionals, National Institutes of Health.

3. Caballero B, Cousins RJ, Tucker KL, Ziegler TR, eds. Modern Nutrition in Health and Disease. 11th ed. Baltimore, MD: Lippincott Williams & Wilkins; 2014:305-16.

4. Olorunnisola Olubukola Sinbad, Ajayi Ayodeji Folorunsho, Okeleji Lateef Olabisi, Oladipo Abimbola Ayoola, Emorioloye Johnson Temitope. Vitamins as Antioxidants. Journal of Food Science and Nutrition Research 2 (2019): 214-235.

5. Vitamin and its importance. Drug Information Centre – Gujarat State Pharmacy Council.

6. Vitamin A and Carotenoids - Health Professional Fact Sheet - National Institues of Health.

7. NUTRITION LANDSCAPE INFORMATION SYSTEM (NLiS) Nutrition and nutrition-related health and development data – World Health Organisation (WHO).

References

8. Huang Z, Liu Y, Qi G, Brand D, Zheng SG. Role of Vitamin A in the Immune System. J Clin Med. 2018 Sep 6;7(9):258.

9. Clagett-Dame M, Knutson D. Vitamin A in reproduction and development. Nutrients. 2011 Apr;3(4):385-428.

10. Capriello S, Stramazzo I, Bagaglini MF, Brusca N, Virili C, Centanni M. The relationship between thyroid disorders and Vitamin A.: A narrative minireview. Front Endocrinol (Lausanne). 2022 Oct 11;13:968215.

11. Zimmermann MB, Jooste PL, Mabapa NS, Schoeman S, Biebinger R, Mushaphi LF, Mbhenyane X. Vitamin A supplementation in iodine-deficient African children decreases thyrotropin stimulation of the thyroid and reduces the goiter rate. Am J Clin Nutr. 2007 Oct;86(4):1040-4.

12. Timoneda J, Rodríguez-Fernández L, Zaragozá R, Marín MP, Cabezuelo MT, Torres L, Viña JR, Barber T. Vitamin A Deficiency and the Lung. Nutrients. 2018 Aug 21;10(9):1132.

13. da Cunha MSB, Campos Hankins NA, Arruda SF. Effect of Vitamin A supplementation on iron status in humans: A systematic review and meta-analysis. Crit Rev Food Sci Nutr. 2019;59(11):1767-1781.

14. F.G. Huffman, Z.C. Shah. Encyclopedia of Food Sciences and Nutrition (Second Edition), 2003

References

15. Underwood BA. The Role of Vitamin A in child Growth, development and Survival. Adv Exp Med Biol. 1994;352:201-8. doi: 10.1007/978-1-4899-2575-6_16.

16. Yee MMF, Chin KY, Ima-Nirwana S, Wong SK. Vitamin A and Bone Health: A Review on Current Evidence. Molecules. 2021 Mar 21;26(6):1757. doi: 10.3390/molecules26061757.

17. Polcz ME, Barbul A. The Role of Vitamin A in Wound Healing. Nutr Clin Pract. 2019 Oct;34(5):695-700.

18. Elsa C Muñoz and others, Iron and zinc supplementation improves indicators of Vitamin A status of Mexican preschoolers, The American Journal of Clinical Nutrition, Volume 71, Issue 3, March 2000, Pages 789–794

19. Li Y, Wei CH, Xiao X, Green MH, Ross AC. Perturbed Vitamin A Status Induced by Iron Deficiency Is Corrected by Iron Repletion in Rats with Pre-existing Iron Deficiency. J Nutr. 2020 Jul 1;150(7):1989-1995. doi: 10.1093/jn/nxaa108.

20. Hodge C, Taylor C. Vitamin A Deficiency. [Updated 2023 Jan 2]. In: StatPearls [Internet]. Treasure Island (FL): StatPearls Publishing; 2023 Jan-. Available from: https://www.ncbi.nlm.nih.gov/books/NBK567744/

21. Palace VP, Khaper N, Qin Q, Singal PK. Antioxidant potentials of Vitamin A and carotenoids

and their relevance to heart disease. Free Radic Biol Med. 1999 Mar;26(5-6):746-61.

22. Murat Gürbüz, Şule Aktaç, Understanding the role of Vitamin A and its precursors in the immune system, Nutrition Clinique et Métabolisme, Volume 36, Issue 2, 2022, Pages 89-98, ISSN 0985-0562.

23. Carazo A, Macáková K, Matoušová K, Krčmová LK, Protti M, Mladěnka P. Vitamin A Update: Forms, Sources, Kinetics, Detection, Function, Deficiency, Therapeutic Use and Toxicity. Nutrients. 2021 May 18;13(5):1703. doi: 10.3390/nu13051703.

24. Huang Z, Liu Y, Qi G, Brand D, Zheng SG. Role of Vitamin A in the Immune System. J Clin Med. 2018 Sep 6;7(9):258.

25. Makita, T., Hernandez-Hoyas, G., Chen, T. H.-P., Wu, H., Rothenberg, E.V., and Sucov. A developmental transition in definitive erythropoiesis: erythropoietin expression is sequentially regulated by retinoic acid receptors and HNF4. H.M. (2001). Genes & Development, April 1, 2001.

26. Capriello S, Stramazzo I, Bagaglini MF, Brusca N, Virili C, Centanni M. The relationship between thyroid disorders and Vitamin A.: A narrative minireview. Front Endocrinol (Lausanne). 2022 Oct 11;13:968215.

27. Farhangi MA, Keshavarz SA, Eshraghian M, Ostadrahimi A, Saboor-Yaraghi AA. The effect of Vitamin A supplement on thyroid function in

premenopausal women. J Am Coll Nutr. 2012 Aug;31(4):268-74.

28. VanBuren CA, Everts HB. Vitamin A in Skin and Hair: An Update. Nutrients. 2022 Jul 19;14(14):2952.

29. Pozniakov SP. Mechanism of action of Vitamin A on cell differentiation and function]. Ontogenez. 1986 Nov-Dec;17(6):578-86.

30. Shoya Iwanami, Shingo Iwami. Encyclopedia of Bioinformatics and Computational Biology, 2019.

31. Clagett-Dame M, Knutson D. Vitamin A in reproduction and development. Nutrients. 2011 Apr;3(4):385-428.

32. Pavlović, Dragan & Markišić, Maja & Bozic, Marija. (2014). Vitamin A and the nervous system. Archives of Biological Sciences. 66. 1585-1590. 10.2298/ABS1404585P.

33. Sajovic J, Meglič A, Glavač D, Markelj Š, Hawlina M, Fakin A. The Role of Vitamin A in Retinal Diseases. Int J Mol Sci. 2022 Jan 18;23(3):1014. doi: 10.3390/ijms23031014.

34. Wilhelm Stahl, Helmut Sies. Chapter 20 - Nutritional protection against photooxidative stress in human skin and eye. Academic Press, 2020, Pages 389-40.

35. Kim JA, Jang JH, Lee SY. An Updated Comprehensive Review on Vitamin A and

Carotenoids in Breast Cancer: Mechanisms, Genetics, Assessment, Current Evidence, and Future Clinical Implications. Nutrients. 2021 Sep 10;13(9):3162.

36. Khoo HE, Ng HS, Yap WS, Goh HJH, Yim HS. Nutrients for Prevention of Macular Degeneration and Eye-Related Diseases. Antioxidants (Basel). 2019 Apr 2;8(4):85. doi: 10.3390/antiox8040085.

37. Ram Reifen. Vitamin A as an anti-inflammatory agent. Proceedings of the Nutrition Society (2002), 61, 397–400 DOI:10.1079/PNS2002172.

38. Kawata A, Murakami Y, Suzuki S, Fujisawa S. Anti-inflammatory Activity of β-Carotene, Lycopene and Tri-n-butylborane, a Scavenger of Reactive Oxygen Species. In Vivo. 2018 Mar-Apr;32(2):255-264. doi: 10.21873/invivo.11232.

39. Cheng J, Balbuena E, Miller B, Eroglu A. The Role of β-Carotene in Colonic Inflammation and Intestinal Barrier Integrity. Front Nutr. 2021 Sep 27;8:723480. doi: 10.3389/fnut.2021.723480.

40. Blaner WS, Shmarakov IO, Traber MG. Vitamin A and Vitamin E: Will the Real Antioxidant Please Stand Up? Annu Rev Nutr. 2021 Oct 11;41:105-131. doi: 10.1146/annurev-nutr-082018-124228. Epub 2021 Jun 11.

41. Yakıncı, Ömer & Süntar, Ipek. (2022). Vitamin A. 10.1016/B978-0-12-819096-8.00064-1.

42. Christophe Antille, Christian Tran, Olivier Sorg, Pierre Carraux, Liliane Didierjean, Jean-Hilaire Saurat. Vitamin A Exerts a Photoprotective Action in Skin by Absorbing Ultraviolet B Radiation. Journal of Investigative Dermatology,Volume 121, Issue 5, 2003, Pages 1163-1167, ISSN 0022-202X.

43. Fiedor J, Burda K. Potential role of carotenoids as antioxidants in human health and disease. Nutrients. 2014 Jan 27;6(2):466-88. doi: 10.3390/nu6020466.

44. Polcz ME, Barbul A. The Role of Vitamin A in Wound Healing. Nutr Clin Pract. 2019 Oct;34(5):695-700.

45. Debreceni B, Debreceni L. Role of vitamins in cardiovascular health and disease. Research Reports in Clinical Cardiology. 2014;5:283-295

46. Zasada M, Budzisz E. Retinoids: active molecules influencing skin structure formation in cosmetic and dermatological treatments. Postepy Dermatol Alergol. 2019 Aug;36(4):392-397.

47. Sweet potato, raw, unprepared (Includes foods for USDA's Food Distribution Program) - US Department of Agriculture - Agricultural Research Service.

48. Khoo HE, Azlan A, Tang ST, Lim SM. Anthocyanidins and anthocyanins: colored pigments as food, pharmaceutical ingredients, and the potential health benefits. Food Nutr Res. 2017 Aug 13;61(1):1361779.

49. Wu K, Erdman JW Jr, Schwartz SJ, Platz EA, Leitzmann M, Clinton SK, DeGroff V, Willett WC, Giovannucci E. Plasma and dietary carotenoids, and the risk of prostate cancer: a nested case-control study. Cancer Epidemiol Biomarkers Prev. 2004 Feb;13(2):260-9. doi: 10.1158/1055-9965.epi-03-0012.

50. Kale raw - US Department of Agriculture - Agricultural Research Service.

51. Peppers sweet red raw - US DEPARTMENT OF AGRICULTURE Agricultural Research Service.

52. Pumpkin, raw - US DEPARTMENT OF AGRICULTURE Agricultural Research Service.

53. Rosca MG, Vazquez EJ, Kern TS, Hoppel CL. Oxidation of fatty acids is source of increased mitochondrial reactive oxygen species production in kidney cortical tubules in early diabetes. Diabetes. 2012 Aug;61(8):2074-83. Epub 2012 May 14.

54. Aprioku JS. Pharmacology of free radicals and the impact of reactive oxygen species on the testis. J Reprod Infertil. 2013 Oct;14(4):158-72.

55. Koh ES, Kim SJ, Yoon HE, Chung JH, Chung S, Park CW, Chang YS, Shin SJ. Association of blood manganese level with diabetes and renal dysfunction: a cross-sectional study of the Korean general population. BMC Endocr Disord. 2014 Mar 8;14:24. doi: 10.1186/1472-6823-14-24.

56. Jandacek RJ. Linoleic Acid: A Nutritional Quandary. Healthcare (Basel). 2017 May 20;5(2):25. doi: 10.3390/healthcare5020025.

57. Oil, rice bran - US DEPARTMENT OF AGRICULTURE Agricultural Research Service.

58. Sheikh FS, Iyer RR. The effect of oil pulling with rice bran oil, sesame oil, and chlorhexidine mouth rinsing on halitosis among pregnant women: A comparative interventional study. Indian J Dent Res 2016;27:508-12.

59. Oil, cottonseed, salad or cooking - US Department of Agriculture. Agricultural Research Service.

60. Al Senaidy AM. Serum vitamin A and beta-carotene levels in children with asthma. J Asthma. 2009 Sep;46(7):699-702. doi: 10.1080/02770900903056195.

61. Hwang JH, Lim SB. Antioxidant and anticancer activities of broccoli by-products from different cultivars and maturity stages at harvest. Prev Nutr Food Sci. 2015 Mar;20(1):8-14.

62. Wang T, Liu YY, Wang X, Yang N, Zhu HB, Zuo PP. Protective effects of octacosanol on 6-hydroxydopamine-induced Parkinsonism in rats via regulation of ProNGF and NGF signaling. Acta Pharmacol Sin. 2010 Jul;31(7):765-74.

63. Lee S, Choi Y, Jeong HS, Lee J. Effect of cooking methods on the content of vitamins and true

retention in selected vegetables. Food Sci Biotechnol. 2017 Dec 12;27(2):333-342.

64. Dasgupta S, Ray SK. Diverse Biological Functions of Sphingolipids in the CNS: Ceramide and Sphingosine Regulate Myelination in Developing Brain but Stimulate Demyelination during Pathogenesis of Multiple Sclerosis. J Neurol Psychol. 2017 Dec;5(1):10.13188/2332-3469.1000035.

65. Wishart DS, Feunang YD, Guo AC, Lo EJ, Wilson M. DrugBank 5.0: a major update to the DrugBank database for 2018. Nucleic Acids Res. 2017 Nov 8.

66. Khatun H, Rahman A, Biswas M, Islam AU. Water-soluble Fraction of Abelmoschus esculentus L Interacts with Glucose and Metformin Hydrochloride and Alters Their Absorption Kinetics after Coadministration in Rats. ISRN Pharm. 2011;2011:260537. doi: 10.5402/2011/260537

67. García-Casal MN, Layrisse M, Solano L, Barón MA, Arguello F, Llovera D, Leets I, Tropper E. Vitamin A and beta-carotene can improve nonheme iron absorption from rice, wheat and corn by humans. J Nutr. 1998 Mar;128(3):646-50. doi: 10.1093/jn/128.3.646.

68. Gabriel F, Suen, Marchini JS, Dutra de Oliveira. High doses of vitamin A impair iron absorption. Nutrition and Dietary Supplements. 2012;4:61-65.

69. Iqbal TH, Lewis KO, Cooper BT. Phytase activity in the human and rat small intestine. Gut. 1994 Sep;35(9):1233-6. doi: 10.1136/gut.35.9.1233.

70. Vitamin A and Iron Interactions - International Vitamin A Consultative Group (IVACG).

71. Christian P, West KP Jr. Interactions between zinc and vitamin A: an update. Am J Clin Nutr. 1998 Aug;68(2 Suppl):435S-441S. doi: 10.1093/ajcn/68.2.435S.

ABOUT THE AUTHOR

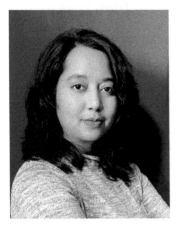

With a Master's Degree in Pharmacy, the author La Fonceur is a Research Scientist and Registered Pharmacist. She specialized in Pharmaceutical Technology and worked as a research scientist in the pharmaceutical research and development department. She is a health blogger and a dance artist. Her previous books include Eat to Prevent and Control Disease, Secret of Healthy Hair, and Eat So What! series. Being a research scientist, she has worked closely with drugs and based on her experience, she believes that one can prevent most of the diseases with nutritious vegetarian foods and a healthy lifestyle.

READ MORE FROM LA FONCEUR

English Editions	Hindi Editions
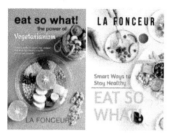 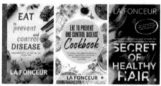	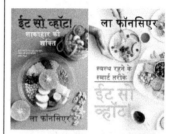 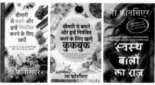

CONNECT WITH LA FONCEUR

Instagram: @la_fonceur | @eatsowhat

Facebook: LaFonceur | eatsowhatblog

Twitter: @la_fonceur

Follow on Bookbub: @eatsowhat

Sign up to get exclusive offers on La Fonceur books:

Blog: http://www.eatsowhat.com/

Website: http://www.lafonceurbooks.com/

COLOR YOUR VITAMIN A

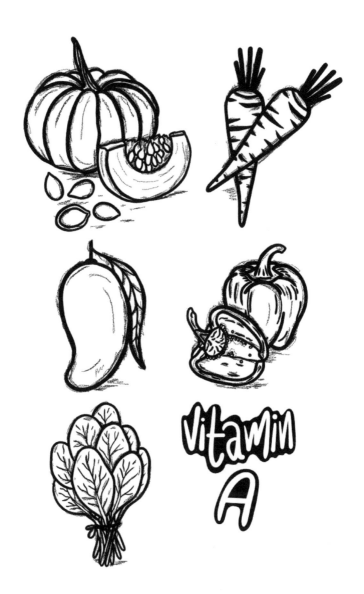

Milton Keynes UK
Ingram Content Group UK Ltd.
UKHW020937220424
441551UK00019B/1409